THE AGING REMEDIES

RECIPES COOKBOOK

Reliable and Confirmed Meal Guide with 30 Delightful Recipes To Having A Healthier Look and Long Lasting Youthful Skin.

SAMMY DAVIDS

Copyright © 2024 by Sammy Davids

All rights reserved.

No part of this publication may be reproduced, distributed, or transmitted in any form or by any means, including photocopying, recording, or other electronic or mechanical methods, without the prior written permission of the publisher, except in the case of brief quotations embodied in critical reviews and certain other noncommercial uses permitted by copyright law.

TABLE OF CONTENTS

4

INTRODUCTION

In our everyday lives, we're often reminded of the passage of time. It's natural to wonder about the secrets to maintaining that youthful glow, to resist the signs of aging that inevitably touch us all. Yet, amidst the chaos of our days, could the answers be as simple as the meals we prepare?

Step into the kitchen, where the vibrant colors of fresh produce beckon. Here, amidst the comforting scents of herbs and spices, we embark on a culinary journey that promises more than just a delicious meal—it offers a way to nourish our skin from within.

With every slice of berry, we're tapping into nature's Vitamin C, a boost of radiance for our skin. The dark, leafy greens offer up Vitamin A, whispering promises of renewal and revitalization.

As we mix and blend, there's a sense of intuition guiding us, an innate knowledge of what our bodies crave. The nuts and seeds, packed with Vitamin E, hint at protection and resilience against time's march.

In these moments of creation, we become alchemists of our own well-being. Each dish is not just a meal; it's a potion of vitality, a blend of flavors and nutrients that speak to our skin's deepest needs.

5

With every savory bite, we feel a surge of energy, as if our skin is awakening to the nourishment it craves. These dishes aren't just about satisfying hunger; they're about feeding our skin's hunger for youth and vibrancy.

In this dance of ingredients and intuition, we uncover the magic of anti-aging. It's not about complex potions or elusive secrets—it's about the simple act of cooking with love and intention. And with each nourishing meal, we take a step towards a future where age is but a number, and our skin glows with timeless vitality.

DELICIOUS ANTI-AGING RECIPES

1. Grilled Salmon with Asparagus

- Ingredients:
    - 4 salmon fillets
    - 1 bunch asparagus, trimmed
    - Olive oil
    - Lemon juice
    - Salt and pepper to taste
- Instructions:
    - Preheat grill to medium-high heat.
    - Brush salmon fillets and asparagus with olive oil and lemon juice.
    - Season with salt and pepper.
    - Grill salmon for 4-5 minutes per side, until cooked through.
    - Grill asparagus for 3-4 minutes, until tender.
    - Serve salmon over asparagus with a squeeze of fresh lemon juice.

- **Nutritional Benefits**

- **Salmon:**
    - Omega-3s: Reduce inflammation, keep skin elastic.
    - Astaxanthin: Protects from UV damage, improves texture.
    - Protein: Supports firm, youthful skin.

7

- **Asparagus**:
    - Antioxidants: Repair and slow down skin aging.
    - Folate: Helps regenerate cells, aids in repair.
    - Vitamin K: Reduces dark circles, evens skin tone.

Anti-Aging Benefits:

1. **Reduce Inflammation**: Omega-3s combat skin inflammation.
2. **UV Protection**: Astaxanthin shields from sun damage.
3. **Firm Skin**: Protein maintains skin elasticity.
4. **Hydrated Skin**: Omega-3s keep skin moisturized.
5. **Cell Renewal**: Folate aids in repairing skin cells.
6. **Radiant Complexion**: Vitamin K promotes glowing skin.
7. **Smooth Skin**: Antioxidants fight fine lines and wrinkles.

8

2. Kale and Quinoa Salad

- **Ingredients**:
  - 2 cups cooked quinoa
  - 4 cups kale, stems removed and chopped
  - 1/2 cup cherry tomatoes, halved
  - 1/4 cup feta cheese, crumbled
  - 1/4 cup walnuts, chopped
  - Lemon vinaigrette (olive oil, lemon juice, Dijon mustard, honey)

- **Instructions**:
  - In a large bowl, combine quinoa, kale, cherry tomatoes, feta, and walnuts.
  - Toss with lemon vinaigrette.
  - Serve chilled as a refreshing and nutrient-packed salad.

- **Nutritional Benefits**

- **Kale**:
  - **Antioxidants**: Fight free radicals, reduce signs of aging.
  - **Vitamin C**: Boosts collagen production for firm skin.
  - **Vitamin K**: Reduces dark circles and promotes skin health.
  - **Iron**: Supports oxygenation of skin cells, improving complexion.

9

- **Quinoa**:
    - **Complete Protein**: Supports muscle and skin tissue repair.
    - **Fiber**: Aids in digestion, promotes clear skin.
    - **Vitamins B & E**: Improve skin elasticity and hydration.
    - **Antioxidants**: Protect skin from environmental damage.

Anti-Aging Benefits:

1. **Antioxidant Power**: Kale's antioxidants combat aging free radicals.
2. **Collagen Boost**: Vitamin C from kale promotes firm, elastic skin.
3. **Skin Repair**: Quinoa's protein aids in cell and tissue repair.
4. **Hydrated Skin**: Fiber and vitamins keep skin moisturized.
5. **Brighter Complexion**: Vitamin K reduces dark circles and evens skin tone.
6. **Wrinkle Reduction**: Antioxidants from quinoa fight fine lines.
7. **Improved Texture**: Iron and vitamins promote smooth, youthful skin.

10

3. Avocado Toast with Poached Eggs

- **Ingredients**:
  - 2 slices whole grain bread, toasted
  - 1 ripe avocado, mashed
  - 2 eggs
  - Salt, pepper, red pepper flakes
  - Optional toppings: cherry tomatoes, microgreens, feta cheese
- **Instructions**:
  - Spread mashed avocado on toasted bread slices.
  - Poach eggs to desired doneness.
  - Place poached eggs on top of avocado toast.
  - Add pepper, salt, and red pepper flakes for seasoning.
  - Garnish with toppings if desired.

- **Nutritional benefits**

- **Avocado**:
  - **Healthy Fats**: Omega-9 fatty acids nourish and hydrate the skin.
  - **Vitamin E**: Powerful antioxidant that protects against skin damage.
  - **Vitamin C**: Boosts collagen production for firm, youthful skin.
  - **Carotenoids**: Reduce wrinkles and improve skin tone.

11

- **Poached Eggs**:
    - **Protein**: Supports collagen synthesis and skin repair.
    - **Biotin**: Promotes healthy hair, skin, and nails.
    - **Vitamin D**: Supports skin cell growth and repair.

Anti-Aging Benefits:

1. **Skin Hydration**: Avocado's healthy fats keep skin supple and moisturized.
2. **Antioxidant Protection**: Vitamin E shields against UV damage and free radicals.
3. **Collagen Boost**: Vitamin C stimulates collagen production for firm skin.
4. **Wrinkle Reduction**: Carotenoids improve skin elasticity and reduce wrinkles.
5. **Tissue Repair**: Protein from eggs aids in skin cell regeneration.
6. **Healthy Skin, Hair, and Nails**: Biotin promotes overall skin health.
7. **Cell Regeneration**: Vitamin D supports the growth of new, healthy skin cells.

4. Blueberry Oatmeal Smoothie

- **Ingredients**:
  - 1/2 cup rolled oats
  - 1/2 cup blueberries
  - 1 banana
  - 1 cup almond milk
  - 1 tablespoon honey
  - 1/2 teaspoon cinnamon
- **Instructions**:
  - Blend all ingredients until smooth.
  - Serve immediately as a nutritious and filling breakfast smoothie.

- **Nutritional benefits**

- **Blueberries**:
  - **Antioxidants**: Combat free radicals, slow down aging.
  - **Vitamin C**: Boosts collagen production, maintains skin elasticity.
  - **Anthocyanins**: Protect against UV damage and improve skin texture.
  - **Fiber**: Supports gut health, aiding in toxin removal.
- **Oats**:
  - **Beta-Glucans**: Reduce inflammation, promote skin healing.
  - **Silica**: Boosts collagen production for fim, plump skin.

13

- **Vitamin E**: Protects skin from oxidative stress, improves moisture retention.
- **Greek Yogurt**:
  - **Protein**: Supports collagen synthesis and skin repair.
  - **Probiotics**: Maintain gut health, improving skin complexion.
  - **Calcium**: Essential for skin cell renewal and regeneration.

Anti-Aging Benefits:

1. **Powerful Antioxidants**: Blueberries' antioxidants fight oxidative stress and slow aging.
2. **Collagen Boost**: Vitamin C and silica promote firm, elastic skin.
3. **UV Protection**: Anthocyanins shield against UV damage and photoaging.
4. **Skin Healing**: Beta-glucans from oats aid in skin repair and regeneration.
5. **Moisture Retention**: Vitamin E locks in moisture for hydrated, plump skin.
6. **Gut Health**: Probiotics support a healthy gut microbiome, reflecting in clear skin.
7. **Cell Renewal**: Calcium supports the turnover of new skin cells for a youthful glow.

5. Greek Yogurt Parfait with Berries

- Ingredients:
    - 1 cup Greek yogurt
    - 1/2 cup mixed berries (strawberries, blueberries, raspberries)
    - 1/4 cup granola
    - Drizzle of honey
- Instructions:
    - Arrange granola, Greek yogurt, and berries in a glass.
    - Repeat layers.
    - Drizzle with honey.
    - Serve chilled as a healthy and satisfying parfait.

- **Nutritional benefits**

- **Greek Yogurt**:
    - **Protein**: Supports collagen synthesis for firm, youthful skin.
    - **Probiotics**: Maintain a healthy gut microbiome, improving skin health.
    - **Calcium**: Essential for skin cell renewal and regeneration.
    - **Vitamin B12**: Promotes cell growth and repair.
- **Berries**:
    - **Antioxidants**: Fight free radicals, slow down skin aging.
    - **Vitamin C**: Boosts collagen production, maintains skin elasticity.

15

- **Anthocyanins**: Protect against UV damage and improve skin texture.
- **Fiber**: Supports gut health, aiding in toxin removal.

Anti-Aging Benefits:

1. **Collagen Support**: Greek yogurt's protein promotes firm, elastic skin.
2. **Gut Health**: Probiotics maintain a healthy gut microbiome, reflecting in clear skin.
3. **Skin Renewal**: Calcium supports the turnover of new skin cells for a youthful glow.
4. **Antioxidant Power**: Berries' antioxidants combat oxidative stress and slow aging.
5. **UV Protection**: Anthocyanins shield against UV damage and photoaging.
6. **Collagen Boost**: Vitamin C from berries promotes firm, plump skin.
7. **Digestive Support**: Fiber aids in toxin removal, promoting clearer skin.

6. Turkey and Veggie Stir-Fry

- **Ingredients**:
    - 1 lb. turkey breast, thinly sliced
    - 2 cups of mixed veggies, such as broccoli, snap peas, and bell peppers
    - 2 cloves garlic, minced
    - 1 tablespoon ginger, grated
    - 1/4 cup low-sodium soy sauce
    - 2 tablespoons olive oil
    - Cooked brown rice
- **Instructions**:
    - In a large skillet or wok, heat the olive oil over medium-high heat.
    - Add turkey slices and stir-fry until browned.
    - Stir-fry the ginger and garlic for one minute.
    - Add mixed vegetables and soy sauce, stir-fry until vegetables are tender-crisp.
    - Serve over cooked brown rice.

- **Nutritional benefits**

- **Turkey**:
    - **Lean Protein**: Supports collagen synthesis for firm, youthful skin.
    - **Selenium**: Protects skin cells from damage and oxidative stress.
    - **Zinc**: Promotes skin repair and regeneration.
    - **Vitamin B6**: Supports cell renewal and overall skin health.

17

- **Mixed Vegetables**:
    - **Antioxidants**: Fight free radicals, slow down skin aging.
    - **Vitamins A and C**: Boost collagen production, maintain skin elasticity.
    - **Fiber**: Supports gut health, aids in toxin removal.
- **Garlic and Ginger**:
    - **Anti-Inflammatory**: Reduce skin redness and inflammation.
    - **Antioxidants**: Protect against environmental damage and premature aging.

Anti-Aging Benefits:

1. **Collagen Support**: Turkey's protein promotes firm, elastic skin.
2. **Skin Protection**: Selenium and vitamins A, C protect against oxidative stress.
3. **Skin Repair**: Zinc aids in wound healing and skin regeneration.
4. **Cell Renewal**: Vitamin B6 supports the turnover of new skin cells.
5. **Antioxidant Power**: Vegetables' antioxidants combat free radicals, slow aging.
6. **Skin Elasticity**: Vitamins A and C maintain skin's firmness and elasticity.

18

7. **Anti-Inflammatory**: Garlic and ginger reduce skin redness and irritation.

7. *Mango and Shrimp Salad*

- Ingredients:
  - 1 lb. cooked shrimp, peeled and deveined
  - 2 mangoes, peeled and diced
  - 1 cucumber, diced
  - 1/4 cup red onion, finely chopped
  - 1/4 cup cilantro, chopped
  - Juice of 1 lime
  - Salt and pepper to taste
- Instructions:
  - In a large bowl, combine shrimp, mangoes, cucumber, red onion, and cilantro.
  - Squeeze lime juice over the salad.
  - Season with salt and pepper.
  - Toss gently to combine.
  - Serve chilled as a refreshing and tropical salad.

- **Nutritional benefits**

- **Shrimp**:
  - **Protein**: Supports collagen synthesis for firm, youthful skin.
  - **Astaxanthin**: Powerful antioxidant that protects skin from UV damage.
  - **Omega-3 Fatty Acids**: Reduce inflammation and maintain skin elasticity.

20

- **Mango**:
    - **Vitamin C**: Boosts collagen production, maintains skin elasticity.
    - **Vitamin A**: Supports skin cell regeneration and repair.
    - **Antioxidants**: Fight free radicals, slow down skin aging.
    - **Fiber**: Supports gut health, aids in toxin removal.

Anti-Aging Benefits:

1. **Collagen Support**: Shrimp's protein promotes firm, elastic skin.
2. **UV Protection**: Astaxanthin shields against UV damage and photoaging.
3. **Skin Renewal**: Vitamin C and A from mango promote cell regeneration.
4. **Antioxidant Power**: Mango's antioxidants combat free radicals, slow aging.
5. **Skin Elasticity**: Omega-3s maintain skin's firmness and elasticity.
6. **Brighter Skin**: Vitamin K reduces dark circles and promotes radiance.
7. **Cell Regeneration**: Folate and iron aid in repairing and renewing skin cells.

8. Caprese Stuffed Chicken Breast

- **Ingredients**:
    - 4 chicken breasts
    - 1 cup cherry tomatoes, halved
    - 1/2 cup fresh mozzarella, diced
    - 1/4 cup fresh basil leaves, chopped
    - Balsamic glaze
    - Salt and pepper to taste
- **Instructions**:
    - Preheat oven to 375°F (190°C).
    - Make a horizontal incision in each chicken breast to form a pocket.
    - Stuff each chicken breast with cherry tomatoes, mozzarella, and basil.
    - Season with salt and pepper.
    - Stuffed chicken breasts should be put on a baking dish.
    - Bake for 25-30 minutes, until chicken is cooked through.
    - Drizzle with balsamic glaze before serving.

- **Nutritional benefits**

- **Chicken Breast**:
    - **Protein**: Supports collagen synthesis for firm, youthful skin.
    - **Selenium**: Protects skin cells from damage and oxidative stress.

22

- **Tomatoes**:
    - **Lycopene**: Powerful antioxidant for skin protection.
    - **Vitamin C**: Boosts collagen production, maintains elasticity.
- **Fresh Mozzarella**:
    - **Protein**: Supports skin structure and repair.
    - **Calcium**: Essential for skin cell renewal.
- **Basil**:
    - **Antioxidants**: Combat oxidative stress, protect skin.
    - **Vitamin K**: Reduces dark circles, promotes skin health.

Anti-Aging Benefits:

1. **Collagen Support**: Protein helps maintain firm, elastic skin.
2. **UV Protection**: Lycopene shields against sun damage.
3. **Skin Renewal**: Nutrients promote cell turnover and repair.
4. **Antioxidant Power**: Protects skin from free radicals.
5. **Skin Elasticity**: Supports firmness and resilience.
6. **Brighter Skin**: Enhances complexion for a radiant look.
7. **Cell Regeneration**: Supports healthy skin cell growth.

23

9. Quinoa Stuffed Bell Peppers

- Ingredients:
    - 4 bell peppers, halved and seeds removed
    - 1 cup cooked quinoa
    - 1 can black beans, drained and rinsed
    - 1 cup corn kernels
    - 1/2 cup diced tomatoes
    - 1/4 cup chopped cilantro
    - 1 teaspoon cumin
    - Salt and pepper to taste
    - Shredded cheddar cheese (optional)
- Instructions:
    - Preheat oven to 375°F (190°C).
    - In a large bowl, mix together quinoa, black beans, corn, tomatoes, cilantro, cumin, salt, and pepper.
    - Spoon the quinoa mixture into each half of the bell pepper.
    - Top with shredded cheddar cheese if desired.
    - Place stuffed peppers in a baking dish.
    - Cover with foil and bake for 30-35 minutes.
    - Remove foil and bake for an additional 10 minutes until peppers are tender

- Nutritional benefits

- .Quinoa:
    - **Protein**: Supports firm, youthful skin.
    - **Antioxidants**: Fight aging free radicals.

24

- **Vitamins B & E**: Improve skin elasticity.
- **Bell Peppers**:
    - **Vitamin C**: Boosts collagen, maintains elasticity.
    - **Beta-Carotene**: Converts to vitamin A for skin repair.
    - **Antioxidants**: Protect against skin damage.
- **Spinach**:
    - **Iron**: Improves complexion, supports cell renewal.
    - **Vitamin A**: Promotes healthy skin turnover.
- **Tomatoes** (in stuffing):
    - **Lycopene**: Powerful antioxidant for skin protection.
    - **Vitamin C**: Boosts collagen, maintains elasticity.

Anti-Aging Benefits:

1. **Collagen Support**: Quinoa protein maintains skin firmness.
2. **Skin Protection**: Antioxidants fight premature aging.
3. **Skin Renewal**: Vitamins promote healthy skin cells.
4. **Antioxidant Power**: Protects skin from damage.
5. **Skin Elasticity**: Nutrients keep skin firm and resilient.
6. **Brighter Skin**: Enhances skin radiance.
7. **Cell Regeneration**: Supports new, healthy skin growth.

10. Chia Seed Pudding with Berries

- Ingredients:
    - 1/4 cup chia seeds
    - 1 cup almond milk
    - 1 tablespoon honey or maple syrup
    - 1/2 teaspoon vanilla extract
    - Mixed berries for topping
- Instructions:
    - In a bowl, whisk together chia seeds, almond milk, honey, and vanilla extract.
    - With periodic stirring, cover and chill for at least two hours or overnight.
    - Serve topped with mixed berries as a nutritious and fiber-rich pudding.

- **Nutritional benefits**

- **Chia Seeds**:
    - **Omega-3 Fatty Acids**: Reduce inflammation, maintain skin elasticity.
    - **Antioxidants**: Fight free radicals, slow down aging.
    - **Fiber**: Promotes digestion and detoxification.
- **Berries**:
    - **Vitamin C**: Boosts collagen production, maintains skin elasticity.
    - **Antioxidants**: Protect against oxidative stress and skin damage.
    - **Fiber**: Supports gut health, aids in toxin removal.

26

Anti-Aging Benefits:

1. **Skin Elasticity**: Omega-3s from chia seeds maintain firm, youthful skin.
2. **Antioxidant Power**: Berries' antioxidants combat free radicals, slow aging.
3. **Collagen Boost**: Vitamin C promotes collagen production for skin firmness.
4. **Skin Protection**: Antioxidants shield skin from damage and premature aging.
5. **Digestive Support**: Fiber aids in detoxification, promoting clearer skin.
6. **Glowing Skin**: Nutrients promote a radiant and healthy complexion.
7. **Cell Renewal**: Supports the regeneration of new, healthy skin cells.

11. Lemon Garlic Herb Baked Salmon

- **Ingredients**:
    - 4 salmon fillets
    - 2 cloves garlic, minced
    - Zest and juice of 1 lemon
    - 2 tablespoons olive oil
    - 1 tablespoon fresh herbs (such as parsley, dill, or thyme)
    - Salt and pepper to taste
- **Instructions**:
    - Preheat oven to 375°F (190°C).
    - In a small bowl, mix together garlic, lemon zest, lemon juice, olive oil, fresh herbs, salt, and pepper.
    - Arrange the salmon fillets on a parchment paper-lined baking pan.
    - Brush salmon with the lemon herb mixture.
    - Bake the salmon for 12 to 15 minutes, or until it is cooked through.
    - Serve hot with steamed vegetables on the side.

- **Nutritional benefits**

- **Salmon**:

    - **Omega-3 Fatty Acids**: Reduce inflammation, maintain skin elasticity.
    - **Protein**: Supports collagen production for firm, youthful skin.

28

- **Selenium**: Protects skin cells from damage and oxidative stress.
- **Lemon**:
    - **Vitamin C**: Boosts collagen production, maintains skin elasticity.
    - **Antioxidants**: Fight free radicals, slow down aging.
- **Garlic**:
    - **Allicin**: Antioxidant compound that protects against skin damage.
    - **Anti-Inflammatory**: Reduces skin redness and irritation.
- **Herbs** (like parsley or dill):
    - **Antioxidants**: Protect skin from environmental damage.
    - **Vitamins and Minerals**: Support skin health and cell regeneration.

Anti-Aging Benefits:

1. **Omega-3 Fatty Acids**: Maintain skin's firmness and elasticity.
2. **Collagen Support**: Protein promotes youthful, resilient skin.
3. **Antioxidant Power**: Lemon and herbs combat free radicals, slow aging.
4. **Skin Protection**: Selenium shields against UV damage and premature aging.

29

5. **Brighter Skin**: Vitamin C enhances skin radiance and evens tone.
6. **Anti-Inflammatory**: Garlic reduces skin redness and irritation.
7. **Cell Regeneration**: Nutrients support healthy skin cell turnover.

12. Mediterranean Chickpea Salad

- Ingredients:
    - 2 cans chickpeas, drained and rinsed
    - 1 cucumber, diced
    - 1 red bell pepper, diced
    - 1/2 red onion, finely chopped
    - 1/4 cup Kalamata olives, sliced
    - 1/4 cup feta cheese, crumbled
    - 1/4 cup fresh parsley, chopped
    - Juice of 1 lemon
    - 2 tablespoons olive oil
    - Salt and pepper to taste
- Instructions:
    - In a large bowl, combine chickpeas, cucumber, bell pepper, red onion, olives, feta, and parsley.
    - Drizzle with lemon juice and olive oil.
    - Season with salt and pepper.
    - Toss gently to combine.
    - Serve chilled as a refreshing and protein-packed salad.

- **Nutritional benefits**

- **Chickpeas**:
    - **Protein**: Maintains skin firmness.
    - **Fiber**: Promotes digestion and detox.
    - **Antioxidants**: Fight aging free radicals.
- **Tomatoes**:
    - **Lycopene**: Protects skin from UV damage.

31

- **Vitamin C**: Boosts collagen, maintains elasticity.
- **Cucumbers**:
  - **Hydration**: Keeps skin moist and plump.
  - **Silica**: Supports skin's elasticity.
- **Red Onion**:
  - **Quercetin**: Guards against skin damage.
  - **Sulfur Compounds**: Aids skin detox.
- **Feta Cheese**:
  - **Calcium**: Renews skin cells.
  - **Protein**: Repairs skin structure.
  - **Vitamin B12**: Nourishes skin cells.
- **Olives**:
  - **Moisture**: Maintains skin's suppleness.
  - **Antioxidants**: Fights signs of aging.

Anti-Aging Benefits:

1. **Skin Firmness**: Chickpeas' protein keeps skin tight.
2. **UV Protection**: Lycopene shields against sun damage.
3. **Hydrated Skin**: Cucumbers keep skin moist and plump.
4. **Antioxidant Power**: Ingredients fight aging free radicals.
5. **Elasticity Boost**: Silica in cucumbers supports skin's bounce.
6. **Brighter Complexion**: Vitamin C evens out skin tone.

7. **Cell Regeneration**: Nutrients support skin cell
    renewal.

13. Spinach and Berry Salad with Poppy Seed Dressing

- **Ingredients**:
    - 4 cups baby spinach
    - 1 cup mixed berries (strawberries, blueberries, raspberries)
    - 1/4 cup sliced almonds
    - 1/4 cup feta cheese, crumbled
    - Poppy seed dressing
- **Instructions**:
    - In a large bowl, combine baby spinach, mixed berries, sliced almonds, and feta cheese.
    - Drizzle with poppy seed dressing.
    - Toss gently to coat.
    - Serve as a vibrant and antioxidant-rich salad.

- **Nutritional benefits**

- **Spinach**:
    - **Vitamin C**: Boosts collagen production, maintains skin elasticity.
    - **Vitamin A**: Supports skin cell regeneration and repair.
    - **Antioxidants**: Fight free radicals, slow down skin aging.
- **Berries** (like strawberries, blueberries, raspberries):
    - **Vitamin C**: Boosts collagen production, maintains skin elasticity.

- **Antioxidants**: Protect against oxidative stress and skin damage.
  - **Fiber**: Supports gut health, aids in toxin removal.
- **Almonds** (optional):
  - **Vitamin E**: Protects skin from sun damage and premature aging.
  - **Healthy Fats**: Maintain skin's moisture and elasticity.
  - **Antioxidants**: Fight free radicals, promote skin health.
- **Poppy Seed Dressing**:
  - **Vitamin C**: Boosts collagen production, maintains skin elasticity.
  - **Omega-3 Fatty Acids** (if made with flaxseed oil): Reduce inflammation, maintain skin health.

Anti-Aging Benefits:

1. **Collagen Boost**: Spinach and berries' vitamin C promotes firm, elastic skin.
2. **Skin Renewal**: Vitamin A supports healthy skin cell turnover.
3. **Antioxidant Power**: Berries and almonds combat free radicals, slow aging.
4. **Skin Protection**: Vitamin E shields against UV damage and premature aging.

35

5. **Moisture Balance**: Healthy fats from almonds maintain skin's hydration.
6. **Brighter Skin**: Vitamin C evens out skin tone and promotes radiance.
7. **Cell Regeneration**: Nutrients support new, healthy skin cell growth.

36

14. Broccoli and White Bean Soup

- **Ingredients**:
    - 1 tablespoon olive oil
    - 1 onion, chopped
    - 2 cloves garlic, minced
    - 4 cups broccoli florets
    - 1 can white beans, drained and rinsed
    - 4 cups vegetable broth
    - Salt, pepper, thyme to taste
    - Optional: grated Parmesan cheese for garnish
- **Instructions**:
    - Warm up the olive oil in a big pot over medium heat.
    - Add onion and garlic, cooking until softened.
    - Add broccoli florets and white beans, stirring to combine.
    - After adding the vegetable broth, boil the mixture.
    - Cook for 15-20 minutes until broccoli is tender.
    - Puree soup with an immersion blender until it's smooth.
    - Season with salt, pepper, and thyme.
    - If preferred, top hot servings with grated Parmesan cheese.

- **Nutritional benefits**

- **Broccoli**:
    - **Vitamin C**: Boosts collagen production, maintains skin elasticity.
    - **Vitamin K**: Reduces dark circles, promotes skin health.
    - **Antioxidants**: Fight free radicals, slow down skin aging.
- **White Beans**:
    - **Protein**: Supports collagen synthesis for firm, youthful skin.
    - **Fiber**: Promotes digestion and detoxification.
    - **Minerals (like zinc)**: Supports skin repair and regeneration.
- **Garlic**:
    - **Allicin**: Antioxidant compound that protects against skin damage.
    - **Sulfur Compounds**: Support skin's natural detoxification.
- **Onion**:
    - **Quercetin**: Antioxidant that guards against skin damage.
    - **Sulfur Compounds**: Aid in skin detox and renewal.
- **Vegetable Broth**:
    - **Nutrients**: Provide essential vitamins and minerals for skin health.

- **Hydration**: Keeps skin moisturized and supple.

Anti-Aging Benefits:

1. **Collagen Support**: Broccoli and white beans promote firm, elastic skin.
2. **Skin Health**: Vitamins and antioxidants from broccoli and onions.
3. **Antioxidant Power**: Ingredients combat free radicals, slow aging.
4. **Skin Renewal**: Garlic and onion support healthy skin turnover.
5. **Detoxification**: Sulfur compounds aid in skin detox and rejuvenation.
6. **Nutrient Boost**: Vegetable broth provides essential skin-loving nutrients.
7. **Hydration**: Soup helps keep skin moisturized and glowing.

15. Turkey and Spinach Meatballs

- **Ingredients**:
    - 1 lb. ground turkey
    - 1/2 cup breadcrumbs
    - 1/4 cup grated Parmesan cheese
    - 1/4 cup chopped fresh parsley
    - 1 egg
    - 2 cups fresh spinach, chopped
    - Salt and pepper to taste
    - Marinara sauce for serving
- **Instructions**:
    - Preheat oven to 375°F (190°C).
    - In a large bowl, mix together ground turkey, breadcrumbs, Parmesan cheese, parsley, egg, spinach, salt, and pepper.
    - Shape the mixture into meatballs and arrange them on a parchment paper-lined baking sheet.
    - Bake for 20-25 minutes until cooked through.
    - Serve meatballs with marinara sauce for dipping or over whole grain pasta.

- **Nutritional benefits**

- **Ground Turkey**:
    - **Protein**: Supports collagen synthesis for firm, youthful skin.
    - **Selenium**: Protects skin cells from damage and oxidative stress.

40

- **B Vitamins**: Promote cell renewal and overall skin health.
- **Spinach**:
    - **Vitamin C**: Boosts collagen production, maintains skin elasticity.
    - **Vitamin A**: Supports skin cell regeneration and repair.
    - **Iron**: Supports oxygenation of skin cells, improving complexion.
- **Garlic**:
    - **Allicin**: Antioxidant compound that protects against skin damage.
    - **Sulfur Compounds**: Support skin's natural detoxification.
- **Herbs (like parsley or basil)**:
    - **Antioxidants**: Combat oxidative stress, protect skin.
    - **Vitamins and Minerals**: Support skin health and cell renewal.

Anti-Aging Benefits:

1. **Collagen Support**: Turkey's protein promotes firm, elastic skin.
2. **Skin Protection**: Selenium and antioxidants shield against damage.
3. **Skin Renewal**: Vitamins A and C promote healthy cell turnover.

41

4. **Antioxidant Power**: Ingredients combat free radicals, slow aging.
5. **Detoxification**: Sulfur compounds aid in skin detox and rejuvenation.
6. **Iron for Complexion**: Spinach's iron improves skin tone and complexion.
7. **Cell Regeneration**: Nutrients support new, healthy skin growth.

16. Roasted Brussels Sprouts with Balsamic Glaze

- **Ingredients**:
    - 1 lb. Brussels sprouts, trimmed and halved
    - 2 tablespoons olive oil
    - Salt and pepper to taste
    - Balsamic glaze
- **Instructions**:
    - Preheat oven to 400°F (200°C).
    - Add salt, pepper, and olive oil to Brussels sprouts and toss.
    - Arrange in a single layer on a baking sheet.
    - Roast until crispy and caramelized, 25 to 30 minutes.
    - Drizzle with balsamic glaze before serving.

- **Nutritional benefits**

- **Brussels Sprouts**:
    - **Vitamin C**: Boosts collagen production, maintains skin elasticity.
    - **Vitamin K**: Reduces dark circles, promotes skin health.
    - **Antioxidants**: Fight free radicals, slow down skin aging.

43

- **Balsamic Glaze**:
    - **Antioxidants**: Protect against oxidative stress and skin damage.
    - **Polyphenols**: Anti-inflammatory properties for skin health.
- **Olive Oil** (used in roasting):
    - **Healthy Fats**: Maintain skin's moisture and elasticity.
    - **Vitamin E**: Protects skin from sun damage and premature aging.
- **Garlic** (optional):
    - **Allicin**: Antioxidant compound that protects against skin damage.
    - **Sulfur Compounds**: Support skin's natural detoxification.

Anti-Aging Benefits:

1. **Collagen Support**: Brussels sprouts' vitamin C promotes firm, elastic skin.
2. **Skin Health**: Vitamins and antioxidants from Brussels sprouts.
3. **Antioxidant Power**: Balsamic glaze and olive oil combat free radicals.
4. **Skin Protection**: Vitamin E shields against UV damage and aging.
5. **Anti-Inflammatory**: Polyphenols in balsamic glaze reduce skin inflammation.
6. **Detoxification**: Sulfur compounds aid in skin detox and renewal.

44

7. **Glowing Skin**: Nutrients promote a radiant and healthy complexion.

45

17. Sweet Potato and Black Bean Tacos

- **Ingredients:**
    - 2 sweet potatoes, peeled and diced
    - 1 can black beans, drained and rinsed
    - 1 tablespoon olive oil
    - 1 teaspoon chili powder
    - 1/2 teaspoon cumin
    - Salt and pepper to taste
    - Corn tortillas
    - Avocado, salsa, cilantro for topping
- **Instructions:**
    - Preheat oven to 400°F (200°C).
    - Toss sweet potatoes with olive oil, chili powder, cumin, salt, and pepper.
    - Roast for 20 to 25 minutes on a baking pan, or until soft.
    - In a saucepan, warm the black beans over medium heat.
    - Warm corn tortillas.
    - Assemble tacos with sweet potatoes, black beans, avocado, salsa, and cilantro.

- **Nutritional benefits**

- **Sweet Potatoes:**
    - **Vitamin A**: Promotes skin cell turnover, maintains skin health.
    - **Vitamin C**: Boosts collagen production, maintains skin elasticity.

46

- **Beta-Carotene**: Converts to vitamin A for skin repair.
- **Black Beans**:
    - **Protein**: Supports collagen synthesis for firm, youthful skin.
    - **Fiber**: Promotes digestion and detoxification.
    - **Antioxidants**: Fight free radicals, slow down skin aging.
- **Avocado** (optional topping):
    - **Healthy Fats**: Maintain skin's moisture and elasticity.
    - **Vitamin E**: Protects skin from UV damage and premature aging.
- **Cilantro** (used as garnish):
    - **Antioxidants**: Combat oxidative stress, protect skin.
    - **Vitamins and Minerals**: Support skin health and cell renewal.

Anti-Aging Benefits:

1. **Collagen Support**: Sweet potatoes' vitamins A and C promote firm, elastic skin.
2. **Skin Repair**: Beta-carotene from sweet potatoes aids in skin cell repair.
3. **Antioxidant Power**: Black beans and cilantro combat free radicals, slow aging.

47

4. **Digestive Health**: Fiber from black beans promotes detoxification and clear skin.
5. **Skin Moisture**: Avocado's healthy fats maintain skin's hydration and suppleness.
6. **UV Protection**: Vitamin E from avocado shields against sun damage.
7. **Cell Renewal**: Nutrients support new, healthy skin growth.

48

18. Cauliflower Rice Stir-Fry

- **Ingredients**:
    - 1 head cauliflower, grated into rice-like pieces
    - 2 tablespoons sesame oil
    - 1 bell pepper, diced
    - 1 cup snap peas
    - 2 carrots, peeled and grated
    - 2 cloves garlic, minced
    - 2 tablespoons low-sodium soy sauce
    - 1 tablespoon rice vinegar
    - 1 teaspoon ginger, grated
    - Optional: cooked shrimp, chicken, or tofu
- **Instructions**:
    - Heat the sesame oil in a big skillet or wok over medium heat.
    - Add bell pepper, snap peas, carrots, and garlic. Stir-fry for 3-4 minutes.
    - Push vegetables to the side of the pan and add cauliflower rice.
    - Stir-fry for 5-6 minutes until cauliflower is tender.
    - In a small bowl, whisk together soy sauce, rice vinegar, and ginger.
    - Pour sauce over cauliflower rice and vegetables.
    - Add cooked protein if desired.
    - Toss to combine and heat through.

49

- **Nutritional benefits**

- **Cauliflower**:
  - **Vitamin C**: Boosts collagen production, maintains skin elasticity.
  - **Antioxidants**: Fight free radicals, slow down skin aging.
  - **Fiber**: Promotes digestion and detoxification.
- **Vegetables** (like bell peppers, carrots, broccoli):
  - **Vitamin C**: Boosts collagen, maintains skin elasticity.
  - **Vitamin A**: Supports skin cell regeneration and repair.
  - **Antioxidants**: Protect against oxidative stress and skin damage.
- **Protein** (like tofu, chicken, shrimp - optional):
  - **Supports collagen synthesis for firm, youthful skin**.
  - **Amino Acids**: Essential for skin cell repair and renewal.
- **Ginger and Garlic** (used in stir-fry sauce):
  - **Antioxidants**: Protect against skin damage and aging.
  - **Anti-Inflammatory**: Reduces skin redness and irritation.
- **Soy Sauce or Tamari** (used in sauce):
  - **Antioxidants**: Protect against oxidative stress and skin damage.

50

- **Sodium**: Regulates skin hydration and moisture balance.

Anti-Aging Benefits:

1. **Collagen Support**: Cauliflower and protein promote firm, elastic skin.
2. **Skin Health**: Vitamins and antioxidants from vegetables.
3. **Antioxidant Power**: Ginger, garlic, and soy sauce combat free radicals.
4. **Digestive Health**: Fiber from cauliflower promotes detoxification and clear skin.
5. **Amino Acids**: Essential for skin cell repair and renewal.
6. **Anti-Inflammatory**: Ingredients reduce skin redness and irritation.
7. **Moisture Balance**: Sodium in soy sauce maintains skin's hydration.

19. Lentil and Vegetable Soup

- **Ingredients**:
    - 1 cup dried lentils, rinsed
    - 4 cups vegetable broth
    - 1 onion, chopped
    - 2 carrots, diced
    - 2 celery stalks, diced
    - 2 cloves garlic, minced
    - 1 teaspoon cumin
    - 1/2 teaspoon smoked paprika
    - 1 bay leaf
    - Salt and pepper to taste
    - Fresh parsley for garnish
- **Instructions**:
    - In a large pot, combine lentils, vegetable broth, onion, carrots, celery, garlic, cumin, smoked paprika, bay leaf, salt, and pepper.
    - Once the lentils are soft, bring to a boil, lower the heat, and simmer for 25 to 30 minutes.
    - Remove bay leaf and adjust seasoning if needed.
    - Serve hot, garnished with fresh parsley.

- **Nutritional benefits**

- **Lentils**:

    - **Protein**: Supports collagen synthesis for firm, youthful skin.
    - **Fiber**: Promotes digestion and detoxification.
    - **Folate**: Aids in cell regeneration and repair.

- **Vegetables** (like carrots, celery, tomatoes):
  - **Vitamin A**: Supports skin cell regeneration and repair.
  - **Vitamin C**: Boosts collagen production, maintains skin elasticity.
  - **Antioxidants**: Fight free radicals, slow down skin aging.
- **Spinach** (optional):
  - **Vitamin C**: Boosts collagen production, maintains skin elasticity.
  - **Iron**: Supports oxygenation of skin cells, improving complexion.
- **Garlic and Onions** (used in soup base):
  - **Allicin**: Antioxidant compound that protects against skin damage.
  - **Sulfur Compounds**: Support skin's natural detoxification.
- **Vegetable Broth**:
  - **Nutrients**: Provide essential vitamins and minerals for skin health.
  - **Hydration**: Keeps skin moisturized and supple.

Anti-Aging Benefits:

1. **Collagen Support**: Lentils' protein promotes firm, elastic skin.
2. **Skin Health**: Vitamins and antioxidants from vegetables.

3. **Antioxidant Power**: Garlic, onions, and vegetables combat free radicals.
4. **Digestive Health**: Fiber from lentils promotes detoxification and clear skin.
5. **Cell Renewal**: Folate aids in cell regeneration and repair.
6. **Iron for Complexion**: Spinach's iron improves skin tone and complexion.
7. **Hydration**: Vegetable broth keeps skin moisturized and glowing.

54

20. Quinoa and Kale Stuffed Acorn Squash

- **Ingredients**:
    - 2 acorn squash, halved and seeds removed
    - 1 cup cooked quinoa
    - 1 cup kale, chopped
    - 1/2 cup dried cranberries
    - 1/4 cup pecans, chopped
    - 1 tablespoon maple syrup
    - 1/2 teaspoon cinnamon
    - Salt and pepper to taste
- **Instructions**:
    - Preheat oven to 400°F (200°C).
    - Place acorn squash halves cut side down on a baking sheet.
    - Bake for 30-35 minutes until tender.
    - In a large bowl, combine cooked quinoa, kale, cranberries, pecans, maple syrup, cinnamon, salt, and pepper.
    - Spoon quinoa mixture into each acorn squash half.
    - Put the oven back on and continue baking for fifteen more minutes.
    - Serve hot as a hearty and nutritious meal.

- **Nutritional benefits**

- **Quinoa**:
  - **Protein**: Supports collagen synthesis for firm, youthful skin.
  - **Fiber**: Promotes digestion and detoxification.
  - **Iron**: Supports oxygenation of skin cells, improving complexion.
- **Kale**:
  - **Vitamin C**: Boosts collagen production, maintains skin elasticity.
  - **Vitamin A**: Supports skin cell regeneration and repair.
  - **Antioxidants**: Fight free radicals, slow down skin aging.
- **Acorn Squash**:
  - **Vitamin C**: Boosts collagen production, maintains skin elasticity.
  - **Beta-Carotene**: Converts to vitamin A for skin repair and protection.
  - **Fiber**: Supports digestive health and clear skin.
- **Walnuts** (used in stuffing):
  - **Omega-3 Fatty Acids**: Reduce inflammation, promote skin health.
  - **Antioxidants**: Protect against oxidative stress and skin damage.
- **Cranberries** (used in stuffing):

- **Antioxidants**: Combat free radicals, slow down skin aging.
- **Vitamin C**: Boosts collagen, maintains skin elasticity.

Anti-Aging Benefits:

1. **Collagen Support**: Quinoa and kale promote firm, elastic skin.
2. **Skin Repair**: Vitamins A and C from kale and acorn squash.
3. **Antioxidant Power**: Walnuts and cranberries combat free radicals.
4. **Digestive Health**: Fiber from quinoa and squash promotes detoxification.
5. **Iron for Complexion**: Quinoa's iron improves skin tone and clarity.
6. **Omega-3s for Inflammation**: Walnuts reduce skin inflammation and redness.
7. **Vitamin C Boost**: Kale, acorn squash, and cranberries promote glowing skin.

21. Baked Apples with Cinnamon and Walnuts

- **Ingredients**:
    - 4 apples, cored
    - 1/4 cup chopped walnuts
    - 1/4 cup dried cranberries
    - 2 tablespoons maple syrup
    - 1 teaspoon cinnamon
    - 1/4 teaspoon nutmeg
    - Greek yogurt for serving
- **Instructions**:
    - Preheat oven to 375°F (190°C).
    - In a bowl, mix together walnuts, cranberries, maple syrup, cinnamon, and nutmeg.
    - Stuff each cored apple with the walnut mixture.
    - Place stuffed apples in a baking dish.
    - Bake apples for 25 to 30 minutes, or until they are soft.
    - Serve warm with a dollop of Greek yogurt.

- **Nutritional benefits**

- **Apples**:
    - **Vitamin C**: Boosts collagen production, maintains skin elasticity.
    - **Antioxidants**: Fight free radicals, slow down skin aging.
    - **Fiber**: Promotes digestion and detoxification.

- **Cinnamon**:
    - **Antioxidants**: Protect against oxidative stress and skin damage.
    - **Anti-Inflammatory**: Reduces skin inflammation and redness.
    - **Regulates Blood Sugar**: Helps prevent glycation, which ages the skin.
- **Walnuts**:
    - **Omega-3 Fatty Acids**: Reduce inflammation, promote skin health.
    - **Antioxidants**: Protect against oxidative stress and skin damage.
    - **Vitamin E**: Nourishes and protects skin from UV damage.
- **Honey** (optional):
    - **Antioxidants**: Combat free radicals, slow down skin aging.
    - **Moisture**: Hydrates and softens the skin.

Anti-Aging Benefits:

1. **Collagen Support**: Apples' vitamin C promotes firm, elastic skin.
2. **Antioxidant Power**: Cinnamon and walnuts combat free radicals.
3. **Fiber for Detoxification**: Supports clear, radiant skin.
4. **Omega-3s for Inflammation**: Walnuts reduce skin inflammation.

59

5. **Skin Protection**: Vitamin E from walnuts protects against UV damage.
6. **Blood Sugar Regulation**: Cinnamon helps prevent glycation, which ages skin.
7. **Moisture and Softness**: Honey hydrates and softens the skin.

22. Pumpkin and Lentil Curry

- **Ingredients**:
    - 1 tablespoon coconut oil
    - 1 onion, chopped
    - 2 cloves garlic, minced
    - 1 tablespoon grated ginger
    - 2 tablespoons curry powder
    - 1 can pumpkin puree
    - 1 can coconut milk
    - 1 cup red lentils, rinsed
    - Salt and pepper to taste
    - Fresh cilantro for garnish
    - Cooked brown rice for serving
- **Instructions**:
    - In a large pot, heat coconut oil over medium heat.
    - Add onion, garlic, and ginger. Cook until softened.
    - Stir in curry powder and cook for 1 minute.
    - Add pumpkin puree, coconut milk, red lentils, salt, and pepper.
    - After bringing to a simmer, lower the heat, and cover.
    - Cook for 20-25 minutes until lentils are tender.
    - Serve over cooked brown rice, garnished with fresh cilantro.

- **Nutritional benefits**

- **Pumpkin**:
    - **Vitamin A**: Supports skin cell renewal.
    - **Vitamin C**: Boosts collagen production.
    - **Beta-Carotene**: Converts to vitamin A for skin health.
- **Lentils**:
    - **Protein**: Supports firm, youthful skin.
    - **Fiber**: Promotes clear, detoxified skin.
    - **Folate**: Aids in cell repair.
- **Coconut Milk**:
    - **Moisture**: Maintains skin's elasticity.
    - **Vitamin E**: Protects against premature aging.
- **Turmeric**:
    - **Anti-Inflammatory**: Reduces redness.
    - **Antioxidants**: Combat skin damage.
- **Ginger and Garlic**:
    - **Antioxidants**: Protect and rejuvenate skin.
    - **Anti-Aging**: Reduce signs of aging.

Anti-Aging Benefits:

1. **Skin Renewal**: Vitamin A from pumpkin.
2. **Collagen Boost**: Vitamin C from pumpkin.
3. **Detoxification**: Fiber from lentils.
4. **Hydration**: Coconut milk's moisture.
5. **Inflammation Reduction**: Turmeric's power.

6. **Protection**: Antioxidants from spices.
7. **Youthful Glow**: Ginger and garlic's benefits.

63

23. Mushroom and Spinach Stuffed Portobello Mushrooms

- **Ingredients**:
    - 4 large portobello mushrooms, stems removed
    - 2 tablespoons olive oil
    - 2 cloves garlic, minced
    - 2 cups baby spinach
    - 1 cup chopped mushrooms
    - 1/4 cup grated Parmesan cheese
    - Salt and pepper to taste
- **Instructions**:
    - Preheat oven to 375°F (190°C).
    - Place portobello mushrooms on a baking sheet.
    - Heat the olive oil in a pan over medium heat.
    - Add garlic and cook for 1 minute.
    - Add baby spinach and chopped mushrooms, cooking until wilted.
    - Take off the heat and mix in the salt, pepper, and Parmesan cheese.
    - Spoon spinach mixture into each portobello mushroom.
    - Bake mushrooms for 20 to 25 minutes, or until they are soft.
    - Serve hot as a savory and satisfying dish.

64

- **Nutritional benefits**

- **Portobello Mushrooms**:
    - **Vitamin D**: Promotes skin cell growth and repair.
    - **Selenium**: Protects skin from damage and aging.
    - **Antioxidants**: Fight free radicals, slow down skin aging.
- **Spinach**:
    - **Vitamin C**: Boosts collagen production, maintains skin elasticity.
    - **Vitamin A**: Supports skin cell regeneration and repair.
    - **Iron**: Supports oxygenation of skin cells, improving complexion.
- **Mushrooms**:
    - **Beta-Glucans**: Support skin health and immunity.
    - **Copper**: Promotes collagen synthesis and skin elasticity.
    - **Antioxidants**: Protect against skin damage and aging.
- **Garlic and Herbs** (used in stuffing):
    - **Allicin**: Antioxidant compound that protects against skin damage.
    - **Sulfur Compounds**: Support skin's natural detoxification.

Anti-Aging Benefits:

1. **Skin Repair**: Vitamin D from mushrooms.
2. **Collagen Boost**: Vitamin C from spinach.
3. **Skin Regeneration**: Vitamin A from spinach.
4. **Skin Elasticity**: Copper from mushrooms.
5. **Antioxidant Power**: Mushrooms' beta-glucans.
6. **Detoxification**: Garlic and herbs' sulfur compounds.
7. **Protection**: Selenium from portobello mushrooms.

24. Sesame Ginger Glazed Carrots

- **Ingredients**:
  - 1 lb carrots, peeled and sliced
  - 2 tablespoons sesame oil
  - 2 tablespoons soy sauce
  - 1 tablespoon honey
  - 1 tablespoon grated ginger
  - 1 tablespoon sesame seeds
  - Fresh cilantro for garnish
- **Instructions**:
  - Steam or boil carrots until tender-crisp.
  - In a skillet, heat sesame oil over medium heat.
  - Add soy sauce, honey, grated ginger, and sesame seeds.
  - Stir in cooked carrots, tossing to coat.
  - Cook for 2-3 minutes until glazed.
  - Garnish with fresh cilantro before serving.

- **Nutritional benefits**

- **Carrots**:
  - **Vitamin A**: Supports skin cell regeneration and repair.
  - **Vitamin C**: Boosts collagen production, maintains skin elasticity.
  - **Antioxidants**: Fight free radicals, slow down skin aging.
- **Sesame Seeds** (used in glaze):

67

- **Omega-3 Fatty Acids**: Reduce inflammation, promote skin health.
  - **Vitamin E**: Nourishes and protects skin from UV damage.
  - **Antioxidants**: Protect against oxidative stress and skin damage.
- **Ginger** (used in glaze):
  - **Anti-Inflammatory**: Reduces skin inflammation and redness.
  - **Antioxidants**: Protect against skin damage and aging.
- **Honey** (used in glaze):
  - **Antioxidants**: Combat free radicals, slow down skin aging.
  - **Moisture**: Hydrates and softens the skin.

Anti-Aging Benefits:

1. **Skin Repair**: Vitamin A from carrots.
2. **Collagen Boost**: Vitamin C from carrots.
3. **Antioxidant Power**: Sesame seeds combat free radicals.
4. **Omega-3s for Inflammation**: Sesame seeds reduce skin inflammation.
5. **UV Protection**: Vitamin E from sesame seeds.
6. **Anti-Inflammatory**: Ginger reduces skin redness.
7. **Moisture and Softness**: Honey hydrates and softens the skin.

68

25. Cucumber Avocado Soup

- **Ingredients**:
    - 2 large cucumbers, peeled and chopped
    - 1 ripe avocado, peeled and pitted
    - 1/4 cup fresh mint leaves
    - 1/4 cup Greek yogurt
    - 1 clove garlic, minced
    - Juice of 1 lime
    - Salt and pepper to taste
- **Instructions**:
    - In a blender, combine cucumbers, avocado, mint leaves, Greek yogurt, garlic, lime juice, salt, and pepper.
    - Blend until smooth.
    - Place in the fridge to chill for a minimum of one hour.
    - Serve cold as a refreshing and creamy soup.

- **Nutritional benefits**

- **Cucumber**:
    - **Hydration**: Keeps skin supple.
    - **Vitamin C**: Boosts collagen for elasticity.
- **Avocado**:
    - **Healthy Fats**: Maintains skin's moisture.
    - **Vitamin E**: Protects from UV damage.
- **Greek Yogurt**:
    - **Protein**: Supports firm, youthful skin.
    - **Probiotics**: Promote healthy skin from within.

- **Lemon Juice**:
    - **Vitamin C**: Boosts collagen production.
- **Fresh Herbs**:
    - **Antioxidants**: Protect against skin damage.

Anti-Aging Benefits:

1. **Hydration**: Keeps skin moisturized.
2. **Healthy Fats**: Maintains skin elasticity.
3. **Collagen Support**: Protein from Greek yogurt.
4. **Antioxidant Power**: Helps combat free radicals.
5. **UV Protection**: Vitamin E shields from sun damage.
6. **Gut Health**: Probiotics support healthy skin.
7. **Skin Renewal**: Antioxidants promote skin health.

26. Walnut and Beet Salad

- **Ingredients**:
    - 4 cups mixed greens (spinach, arugula, kale)
    - 1 cup roasted beets, diced
    - 1/2 cup walnuts, toasted
    - 1/4 cup crumbled goat cheese
    - Balsamic vinaigrette
- **Instructions**:
    - In a large bowl, combine mixed greens, roasted beets, walnuts, and goat cheese.
    - Drizzle with balsamic vinaigrette.
    - Toss gently to coat.
    - Serve as a colorful and nutrient-rich salad.

- **Nutritional benefits**

- **Walnuts**:
    - **Omega-3 Fatty Acids**: Reduce inflammation, promote skin health.
    - **Vitamin E**: Nourishes and protects skin from UV damage.
    - **Antioxidants**: Protect against oxidative stress and skin damage.
- **Beets**:
    - **Vitamin C**: Boosts collagen production, maintains skin elasticity.
    - **Folate**: Aids in cell regeneration and repair.

71

- **Antioxidants**: Fight free radicals, slow down skin aging.
- **Leafy Greens** (like arugula or spinach - used in salad):
  - **Vitamin A**: Supports skin cell regeneration and repair.
  - **Vitamin K**: Improves skin elasticity and reduces dark circles.
  - **Antioxidants**: Protect against skin damage and aging.
- **Citrus Dressing** (used in salad):
  - **Vitamin C**: Boosts collagen production, maintains skin elasticity.
  - **Antioxidants**: Protect against skin damage and aging.

Anti-Aging Benefits:

1. **Omega-3s for Skin Health**: Walnuts reduce inflammation.
2. **Vitamin E Protection**: Nourishes and protects skin.
3. **Collagen Boost**: Vitamin C from beets and dressing.
4. **Cell Renewal**: Folate aids in cell regeneration.
5. **Antioxidant Power**: Walnuts, beets, and greens combat free radicals.
6. **Skin Elasticity**: Vitamin K from leafy greens.
7. **UV Protection**: Antioxidants shield from sun damage.

72

27. Cauliflower and Broccoli Detox Salad

- Ingredients:
  - 1 head cauliflower, grated
  - 1 head broccoli, grated
  - 1/2 cup dried cranberries
  - 1/4 cup pumpkin seeds
  - 1/4 cup sunflower seeds
  - Lemon tahini dressing
- Instructions:
  - In a large bowl, combine grated cauliflower, broccoli, cranberries, pumpkin seeds, and sunflower seeds.
  - Drizzle with lemon tahini dressing.
  - Toss gently to combine.
  - Serve chilled as a detoxifying and crunchy salad.

- Nutritional benefits

- **Cauliflower**:
  - **Vitamin C**: Boosts collagen for elasticity.
  - **Antioxidants**: Fight free radicals.
- **Broccoli**:
  - **Vitamin A**: Supports skin renewal.
  - **Vitamin K**: Improves skin elasticity.
- **Carrots**:
  - **Beta-Carotene**: Converts to vitamin A.
  - **Antioxidants**: Combat skin aging.
- **Lemon Dressing**:

73

- **Vitamin C**: Boosts collagen production.
  - **Detoxifying**: Supports clear, glowing skin.
- **Pumpkin Seeds**:
  - **Omega-3s**: Reduce inflammation.
  - **Zinc**: Supports skin health.

Anti-Aging Benefits:

1. **Collagen Boost**: Vitamin C from vegetables and dressing.
2. **Skin Renewal**: Vitamin A from broccoli and carrots.
3. **Antioxidant Power**: Vegetables and seeds combat free radicals.
4. **Detoxification**: Supports clear, glowing skin.
5. **Skin Elasticity**: Vitamin K from broccoli.
6. **Omega-3s for Inflammation**: Pumpkin seeds reduce redness.
7. **Zinc for Skin Health**: Supports collagen production.

28. Garlic Lemon Shrimp Skewers

- **Ingredients**:
    - 1 lb. large shrimp, peeled and deveined
    - 3 cloves garlic, minced
    - Zest and juice of 1 lemon
    - 2 tablespoons olive oil
    - Salt and pepper to taste
    - Wooden skewers, soaked in water
- **Instructions**:
    - In a bowl, combine shrimp, garlic, lemon zest, lemon juice, olive oil, salt, and pepper.
    - Marinate for at least 30 minutes.
    - Thread shrimp onto skewers.
    - Set the grill pan or grill to medium-high heat.
    - Grill shrimp skewers for 2-3 minutes per side until pink and cooked through.
    - Serve hot as a flavorful and protein-packed dish.

- **Nutritional benefits**

- **Shrimp**:
    - **Protein**: Supports collagen for elasticity.
    - **Omega-3s**: Reduce inflammation, promote skin health.
    - **Antioxidants**: Protect against skin damage.
- **Garlic** (in marinade):
    - **Antioxidants**: Protects against skin damage.
    - **Detoxifying**: Supports skin's detox process.
- **Lemon** (in marinade):
    - **Vitamin C**: Boosts collagen production.
    - **Antioxidants**: Protect against skin aging.
- **Olive Oil** (in marinade):
    - **Healthy Fats**: Maintains skin's moisture.
    - **Vitamin E**: Protects from UV damage.
- **Fresh Herbs** (like parsley or cilantro):
    - **Antioxidants**: Protect against skin damage.
    - **Vitamins**: Support skin health.

Anti-Aging Benefits:

1. **Collagen Support**: Protein and Omega-3s.
2. **Antioxidant Power**: Garlic, lemon, herbs combat free radicals.
3. **Vitamin C Boost**: Lemon boosts collagen.
4. **Healthy Fats**: Olive oil maintains moisture.
5. **UV Protection**: Vitamin E from olive oil.

76

6. **Detoxification**: Garlic supports skin detox.
7. **Skin Renewal**: Herbs provide vitamins for skin health.

29. Zucchini Noodles with Pesto and Cherry Tomatoes

- Ingredients:
  - 2 large zucchini, spiralized
  - 1/2 cup cherry tomatoes, halved
  - 1/4 cup pesto sauce
  - Parmesan cheese for garnish
  - Pine nuts for garnish
- Instructions:
  - Heat the olive oil in a pan over medium heat.
  - Add cherry tomatoes and cook until softened.
  - Add zucchini noodles and pesto sauce.
  - Coat and cook for 2 to 3 minutes, or until thoroughly cooked.
  - Serve hot, garnished with Parmesan cheese and pine nuts.

- Nutritional benefits

- **Zucchini Noodles**:
  - **Vitamin C**: Boosts collagen for skin elasticity.
  - **Antioxidants**: Fight free radicals, slow down skin aging.
  - **Hydration**: Keeps skin moisturized.
- **Basil Pesto** (used in dish):
  - **Vitamin K**: Improves skin elasticity.
  - **Antioxidants**: Protect against skin damage.
  - **Healthy Fats**: Maintain skin's moisture.

78

- **Cherry Tomatoes**:
    - **Vitamin C**: Boosts collagen production.
    - **Lycopene**: Protects skin from sun damage.
    - **Antioxidants**: Combat free radicals.
- **Garlic** (in pesto):
    - **Antioxidants**: Protect against skin damage.
    - **Sulfur Compounds**: Support skin's detox process.
- **Olive Oil** (in pesto):
    - **Healthy Fats**: Maintain skin's moisture.
    - **Vitamin E**: Protects from UV damage.

Anti-Aging Benefits:

1. **Collagen Boost**: Vitamin C from zucchini and tomatoes.
2. **Antioxidant Power**: Basil, tomatoes combat free radicals.
3. **Vitamin K for Elasticity**: Basil in pesto.
4. **Hydration**: Zucchini keeps skin moisturized.
5. **Lycopene Protection**: Cherry tomatoes guard against sun damage.
6. **Healthy Fats**: Olive oil in pesto maintains moisture.
7. **Detoxification**: Garlic supports skin detox.

30. Coconut Chia Seed Pudding with Berries

- **Ingredients**:
    - 1/4 cup chia seeds
    - 1 cup coconut milk
    - 1 tablespoon honey or maple syrup
    - 1/2 teaspoon vanilla extract
    - Mixed berries for topping
- **Instructions**:
    - In a bowl, whisk together chia seeds, coconut milk, honey, and vanilla extract.
    - With periodic stirring, cover and chill for at least two hours or overnight.
    - Serve topped with mixed berries as a creamy and nutrient-packed pudding.

- **Nutritional benefits**

- **Chia Seeds**:
    - **Omega-3 Fatty Acids**: Reduce inflammation, promote skin health.
    - **Antioxidants**: Protect against oxidative stress and skin damage.
    - **Fiber**: Supports gut health for radiant skin.
- **Coconut Milk** (used in pudding):
    - **Medium-Chain Triglycerides (MCTs)**: Nourish skin from within.
    - **Vitamin E**: Protects from UV damage, promotes skin elasticity.

80

- **Berries** (like strawberries, blueberries, raspberries - used as topping):
  - **Vitamin C**: Boosts collagen production, maintains skin elasticity.
  - **Antioxidants**: Combat free radicals, slow down skin aging.
- **Cinnamon** (used in pudding):
  - **Antioxidants**: Protect against skin damage.
  - **Anti-Inflammatory**: Reduces skin redness and irritation.
- **Maple Syrup** (used for sweetness):
  - **Antioxidants**: Combat oxidative stress, promote skin health.

Anti-Aging Benefits:

1. **Omega-3s for Skin Health**: Chia seeds reduce inflammation.
2. **Healthy Fats**: MCTs from coconut milk nourish skin.
3. **Collagen Boost**: Vitamin C from berries.
4. **Antioxidant Power**: Berries, cinnamon, and maple syrup combat free radicals.
5. **Vitamin E Protection**: Coconut milk shields from UV damage.
6. **Gut Health**: Chia seeds' fiber promotes healthy skin.
7. **Skin Radiance**: Antioxidants promote a youthful complexion

CONCLUSION

In the culinary alchemy of anti-aging recipes, we've uncovered more than just ways to nourish our bodies—we've discovered the key to unlocking timeless vitality. Each dish, crafted with intention and love, is a testament to the power of nature's bounty. As we savor the flavors of berries bursting with Vitamin C, greens rich in Vitamin A, and nuts brimming with Vitamin E, we're not just feeding our hunger; we're feeding our skin's deepest cravings for renewal and resilience. This cookbook isn't just a collection of recipes; it's a guide to a life infused with vibrancy and youthfulness. So let us raise our forks to a future where age is just a number, and our skin glows with the radiance of wellness from within. Here's to embracing the magic of anti-aging, one delicious bite at a time.

HAPPY COOKING WHILE LOOKING FOREVER YOUNG!!!